CARING FOR THE CARER

A GUIDED MEMOIR ON PALLIATIVE CARE, CAREGIVING AND LETTING GO

ANOTHILE DOLO

First Published 2026 by Anothile Dolo

ISBN 978-0-903733-81-6 (Print - Paperback)
ISBN 978-0-903733-80-9 (eBook)

Cover design and interior crafted by the team at
www.myebook.online

For my mother, who taught me how to live honestly.

And how to die without pretending.

CONTENTS

1

December 2014 – The Letter

Every December, we drove home. From Cape Town to Umzinto in KwaZulu-Natal. The twenty-hour drive along long roads, with children restless in the back seat, carried a familiar rhythm; it was an act of returning to where I first learned who I was. It was tradition; no matter how busy work became, no matter how heavy the year, December meant home.

My mother's house always smelled the same: of linen, sunlight on curtains, something faintly floral. By December 2014 she had already been on incapacity leave from teaching for some time. Cancer had slowly reduced her classroom to a memory. The liposarcoma that had begun approximately ten years earlier had returned after treatment, and spread. uMa could no longer work. Every year, I helped her with the required paperwork. Forms. Reports. Submissions. As an occupational therapist, it felt practical to me. Useful. Something I could control.

The day before we were due to drive back to Cape Town, I went to say goodbye.

It was just the two of us in her bedroom.

Bedrooms hold truths that lounges do not. They are the spaces where illness settles. Where fatigue stops pretending. Where dignity sometimes feels fragile.

She handed me an envelope.

"Read this," she said.

Her voice was steady. Too steady.

It was a letter from her specialist. I recognised the format immediately: clinical tone, formal structure, careful phrasing. I began reading as a clinician.

Advanced disease.

Poor prognosis.

Not amenable to curative treatment.

Recommendation: permanent incapacity.

And then the sentence that rearranged the room:

The patient is considered terminal.

I do not remember breathing.

She already knew. Of course she knew; she had read it before I did. She wanted me to know, but she did not want to be the one to say the word.

Terminal.

It's a clinical word, efficient, contained. It does not describe the sound of your mother moving slower. It does not describe the way your throat tightens when you look up from a page and realise time has become measurable.

I lowered the letter. She watched my face.

There are moments in life when roles dissolve. I was no longer a healthcare professional. I was not the efficient daughter organising documents. I was simply a child holding proof that uMa was dying.

Neither of us cried, not then at least.

We sat in the quiet understanding that something irreversible had been named.

I don't remember what we said after I lowered the letter. What I do remember is understanding the psychological game uMa was playing – the careful avoidance and the unspoken agreement to protect each other from what could not be changed. She did not want to say the word. I did not want to let her see what it did to me.

I don't remember comforting her.

That truth has taken years to surface.

Perhaps I was trying to be strong for her. Perhaps I believed that my composure would spare her the pain of watching her illness wound me too. Perhaps, in that moment, strength looked like containment.

What I do remember clearly is her instruction that my siblings were not to know. "Confidentiality," she called it. I understood what it really meant. This knowledge was being entrusted to me because I was the one who could carry it, the one who always had.

So, I carried it.

The letter.

The word.

The future it implied.

I carried it alone.

The next day, I drove back to Cape Town with my family.

From that moment on, I was not only her daughter; I was also the keeper of what was coming.

Reflection: Then and Now

At the time, I believed maintaining that silence was a form of protection – for uMa, for my siblings, and for me. Carrying the truth alone felt like strength. Looking back, I can see how quickly responsibility replaced emotion. I became the keeper of information before I had allowed myself to become the keeper of grief.

Clinical Insight: Receiving a Terminal Diagnosis

Terminal diagnoses are often communicated in fragments, letters, or euphemisms. When families receive this information indirectly, emotional processing may be delayed. In this situation, the initial response is often containment rather than expression.

Caregiver Takeaway

If you are the first to know the diagnosis, know this: carrying the truth alone is heavy. You are allowed to seek support even when others are not ready to hear what you know.

2

January 2015 – Back in Cape Town

The drive back from Umzinto had been strenuous.

My children were five- and two years old back then – small, dependent, and demanding. Somewhere along the journey, my youngest, my son, developed a fever. Two-year-olds generally do not tolerate long distances well, and neither did I.

We stopped at an emergency room along the way. The clinical smells and harsh lighting arrived too soon after the letter I had read the day before. I sat there with a feverish toddler in my arms, acutely aware of how quickly vulnerability can assert itself, and how thin the line is between good health and crisis. You can be going about your day, functioning and well, and then find yourself in a hospital waiting room before you've had time to catch your breath. I did what caregivers do – I managed, soothed, and waited – but the sense of being stretched too far had already begun.

When we finally arrived back in Cape Town, I returned to work. The city received me as it always had: traffic dense with routine, never-ending school demands, and in-boxes filled with tasks that assumed continuity. From the outside, my life appeared intact. On the inside, it was beginning to fracture under the weight of too many unknowns.

At the time, I was working as an occupational therapist within the insurance industry. My role did not involve sitting across from patients or listening to their stories directly; instead, I read reports – volumes of them. Functional assessments. Specialist opinions. Prognostic language carefully crafted to justify occupational incapacity.

The terminology was familiar.

Permanent.

Poor prognosis.

Not fit for work.

I read these words daily, detached enough to make decisions, close enough to recognise their weight. What I did not do was actively listen to patients' voices. My work required analysis, not presence, judgement, not empathy. That distance, I told myself, was a strength.

At home, life demanded just as much regulation. My two young children needed structure and reassurance, whatever challenges arose. Illness passed through the household with the usual relentlessness of early childhood. Sleep was fragmented. Decisions felt constant and unfinished.

At the same time, my marriage stood at the edge of a major transition; my husband had secured a job abroad. The plan was for me and the children to join him, but the move had already been delayed, its timing uncertain. And now, layered on top of that logistical complexity, was the knowledge I had not yet shared fully with my husband – perhaps not even with myself.

uMa was terminal.

I did not know how to reconcile these realities. How could I plan a future elsewhere while preparing for an ending here? How could I justify leaving when I knew what was coming? And how could I stay without resenting the life I was being asked to postpone – or the one I might be leaving behind?

Every option carried loss. Every option cost something.

Professionally, I functioned well. Personally, I deferred decisions. Emotionally, I suspended myself somewhere between roles – mother, wife, daughter, clinician – without allowing any one of them full expression.

And still, I carried the secret, honouring uMa's wish for confidentiality, even as the weight of it settled into something far more personal than professional.

My siblings did not know; the burden of knowledge remained mine alone. I framed it as respect for my mother's wishes, but in truth, it was also avoidance of conversations I did not yet know how to survive.

I told myself there would be a right time. A clearer moment. A point at which the path forward would declare itself.

Instead, what arrived was an accumulation of responsibility, uncertainty, and quiet grief.

Reflection: Then and Now

At the time, I believed I was simply managing a difficult season.

Looking back, I can see how many transitions were converging at once – young children, professional responsibility, marital uncertainty, geographic displacement, and anticipatory grief. None of these alone would have undone me, but together, they demanded a level of emotional endurance I did not acknowledge.

I mistook postponement for stability.

Clinical Insight: Decision Paralysis in Caregivers

When caregivers face multiple competing life transitions, their ability to make decisions often becomes immobilised. This is not indecision; it is cognitive overload.

Caregivers may delay major choices, relocation, career shifts, or family disclosures while waiting for certainty that does not exist. In palliative contexts, this paralysis is often compounded by guilt and loyalty conflicts.

Functioning continues but planning stops.

Caregiver Takeaway

If your life feels suspended between incompatible truths, understand this: it is not a personal failure to struggle with impossible choices. Some decisions cannot be made cleanly. Sometimes the most honest response is to pause and seek support before the weight becomes unmanageable.

3

March 2015 – What She Sounded Like

Over the next few months, uMa's health declined in fragments, not in a straight line or in a way that could be tracked neatly on a chart. Alerts about the decline arrived through phone calls, usually from my eldest sister, Sis' Gugu, often in tears.

"She's back in hospital again."

"She's so weak today."

"I don't know how much longer I can do this."

Each call carried urgency and exhaustion. Sis' Gugu spoke of endless admissions, and of waiting rooms and corridors that blurred into one another. She spoke of strain, the kind that builds surreptitiously, day after day, until the body begins to protest.

She was caring for our mother in real time, absorbing the physical labour and emotional weight of proximity, while I listened from a distance, trying to translate her distress into something I could act on.

And yet, when I phoned uMa, she sounded well.

Her voice carried its familiar confidence – the same warmth, the same ease, the same jokes. She asked about the children and dismissed concern with practised lightness. Over the phone, she was still herself: contained, competent, reassuring.

Distance became a collaborator in denial. I told myself that Sis' Gugu was simply overwhelmed, and that the weight of caregiving had sharpened her perception of decline. I told myself that uMa, the woman I had always known, the one who had endured so much already, would carry herself longer than even I believed possible.

I trusted the voice I wanted to believe.

But the calls from my sister continued.

Eventually, I decided to go home.

In March 2015, I travelled back to Umzinto, telling myself I was going to "check in", to see for myself how she was doing. As a clinician, I understood the importance of first-hand assessment; as a daughter, I still hoped to be reassured.

What I saw was not what I had heard in my calls with my mother. Her body told a different story: weight loss, fatigue etched into her posture, and movements slowed not by choice, but by necessity. She looked smaller, as if the space she occupied in the world had begun to contract.

It was the moment when sound finally surrendered to the reality of sight.

At the hospital, I ran into an old university friend, Nombulelo (Buleh to those who knew her well), who was working as a physiotherapist on the ward.

Buleh and I had met during my first year of study in 2003. She was a little more senior than I was, already finding her footing in the professional student life while I was still trying to understand where I belonged. Over the years, our friendship had settled into something steady and familiar. Buleh had met uMa a few times and knew enough about my life to understand what mattered to me – and what it cost when those things began to unravel.

Now, at the hospital, I suddenly remembered a visit uMa had made to our university residence, R Block, during those early student years. Buleh happened to be there that afternoon, and she and uMa had exchanged brief greetings and laughter in the corridor, the first of what would become several small interactions over the years that followed, highlighting for me the easy humour uMa carried into most rooms. It had been a small moment, almost forgettable at the time, but it lingered with me now.

Buleh and I exchanged greetings in the ward entrance, the easy shorthand of people who shared both professional training and personal history. I had not expected to see her there, and yet there she was, familiar and steady, in a place where nothing else felt either. I cannot fully explain what it stirred in me. Relief, perhaps?

Then she asked a question I had been avoiding: "How are you doing?"

It was not clinical, it was not procedural, it was human.

Something in me gave way.

"uMa is dying," I said. And for the first time, I cried. It wasn't quiet or private; I cried with the kind of grief that arrives when truth is finally spoken aloud. In naming it, I crossed a threshold I had been standing at for months.

It had taken me three months. Three months to stop managing. Three months to stop functioning. Three months to stop believing that preparedness could replace mourning.

In that hospital corridor, I finally became what I had been resisting. I was no longer the clinician; I was not the strong one or the keeper of information. I was just a daughter facing the end of her mother's life.

Reflection: Then and Now

At the time, I believed I was being rational, cautious, measured, emotionally contained. Now I understand that I was grieving in instalments. Distance, professional language, and my mother's carefully maintained voice allowed me to postpone accepting the truth. But grief does not disappear when delayed; it simply waits.

What broke the stalemate was not clinical evidence. It was human recognition, someone asking how *I* was.

Clinical Insight: The Power of Witnessing

Patients nearing the end of their life often preserve emotional normalcy for those they love. Phone calls become performances of reassurance, and caregivers at a distance may cling to these interactions, using them to counter reports of decline.

Denial is not always rejection of the truth; sometimes it is a temporary structure that allows caregivers to keep functioning until they are ready to see.

It's often not information that enables them to accept the reality, but rather *witnessing* – being seen by another person at the moment truth becomes unavoidable.

Caregiver Takeaway

If it takes time for you to name what is happening, you are not failing. Acceptance is not a single moment; it is a process. Sometimes, all it takes is one person asking the right question and being willing to hold the answer.

4

March 2015 – What the File Revealed

Hospitals hold truths that families often do not have access to.

While uMa slept, I read her hospital file. It was not merely out of curiosity; it was necessity. As an occupational therapist, I know how to read between the lines – how to interpret the shorthand, the omissions, and the carefully neutral language that disguises what would otherwise be unbearable.

The chemotherapy had taken its toll. uMa had developed renal failure. Radiation had severely burned through one of her lungs, while cancer had spread to the other. What I had interpreted as fatigue was actually physiological depletion; her body was no longer compensating, it was enduring.

I realised she was in constant pain. Not the episodic discomfort she minimised over the phone, but pain that required regular management, the kind that narrows a life, constricts movement, and makes even rest expensive.

At the time, her only companion was her elderly mother – two frail bodies attempting to care for one another, neither fully capable of providing the other's needs. The reality was unmistakable: this living arrangement was no longer safe.

Decisions had to be made.

I spoke to her doctor, and the conversation was clinical, direct, and without ambiguity: in his opinion, she was not medically fit to travel across provinces, even by air. The physiological stress alone posed significant risk. Movement itself had become dangerous.

The option I had been quietly holding, of taking her back with me, dissolved in that moment.

At the same time, other parts of my life were unravelling.

Work had become intolerable. The cumulative strain of carrying too much for too long had begun to surface physically and emotionally, so I had resigned from my job and was due to start a new one in April. I had no leave available, no margin for collapse.

That same month, my husband was leaving to begin his job abroad.

Everything was shifting at once.

I stood at the intersection of professional knowledge, familial responsibility, and personal fracture, with no configuration that offered relief. I could not stay in KwaZulu-Natal indefinitely. I could not take her with me. I could not pause my own life without consequence.

So I left. Without a plan.

There is a particular kind of grief that accompanies you when you leave someone you love in decline not because you want to, but because you have run out of alternatives. It is not abandonment, although it feels like it. The leaving looked like a decision from the outside. From the inside, however, it never felt like one. I did not choose to leave; I had no choice.

I returned to Cape Town carrying images I could not unsee, information I could not unknow, and a guilt that required no explanation. This time, I did not pretend I was fine.

Reflection: Then and Now

At the time, I believed that better planning would have made the journey easier. The logistics of travelling with and for a seriously ill person across provinces, without always having the financial resources to do it well took a toll. Now I understand that no amount of planning could have reconciled what was really pulling at me. I loved uMa deeply and wanted to be present for her daily, but I was also living in a different province, holding down a full-time job, raising young children, and trying to sustain a marriage under enormous strain. Terminal illness compresses time, but it does not simplify life. I had never truly allowed myself to imagine it. Somewhere beneath the practicalities and the planning, I had held onto the hope that uMa would be cured – that treatment would work, that life would normalise again, that we would one day look back on this as a chapter rather than an ending. Terminal illness does not remove the complexity of living; it adds to it, while quietly removing the luxury of time, and the comfort of hope. It exposes fault lines that already exist – in systems, families, and individuals.

Leaving did not mean I stopped caring, it just meant I had reached the limit of what one person could hold.

Clinical Insight: Moral Distress in Caregivers

Moral distress occurs when individuals know the ethically appropriate action to take but are constrained from taking it. In caregiving, this often arises when personal, professional, and systemic limitations collide. Caregivers may experience guilt, shame, or self-blame, even when no better alternative exists.

Naming moral distress does not remove the pain, but it does at least contextualise it. This is not failure; it is exposure to an impossible situation.

Caregiver Takeaway

If you have had to leave your loved one without a plan, understand this: absence does not equal indifference. Sometimes care looks like implementing the least harmful choice available, even when it still hurts.

5

April–July 2015 – Holding Her from Afar

For the next two months, uMa was in and out of hospital.

Care was shared between Sis' Gugu, my brother (Mpendulo, or Mpe to us), and the domestic helper who tried to keep the household functioning. It was a patchwork of goodwill and exhaustion. None of it was practical or sustainable. Everyone was doing their best, but still, the cracks showed.

Although I was far away physically, I stayed in close contact with uMa's treating doctors. I phoned. I emailed. I requested updated reports. I asked questions that hovered at the edge of feasibility. Would she tolerate travel? What would it take to stabilise her? Could we try?

In the background, my own life continued to unravel.

I had started a new job, but it wasn't going well in my view. Before this season, I had been confident in my work, decisive, competent, consistently recognised as a top performer. I had trusted my clinical judgement. But in this new role, I felt suddenly diminished. Distracted. Unsteady. Not because my skills had disappeared, but because my attention was split in ways I could not reconcile.

I felt as though I was at the bottom of the food chain, even though I knew I was capable.

Rather than hiding my challenges, I chose to be honest with my new employer. Early on, I told them what was happening. I had no leave available, but I also knew I needed to be elsewhere at least some of the time. I could not present this as a temporary inconvenience; uMa was dying, and I was managing her care from another province. There was no formal arrangement, and no paperwork, just a quiet, human understanding that I needed flexibility, and that they would extend it. I was deeply grateful, because it made the impossible slightly more manageable. It also lifted something I had not fully acknowledged I was carrying – the guilt of asking, and the quiet shame of feeling like a senior assessor who was underperforming, despite the reputation that had preceded me. I had arrived with a professional identity, but now grief was quietly dismantling it from the inside

My days became divided. Work hours were punctuated by phone calls to doctors, hospitals and medical aids. I chased referrals, requested reports, and clarified plans that remained provisional at best. Through this stage, for me caregiving looked like administration – quiet, invisible, cognitively relentless.

In July, I went home again. uMa's deterioration was unmistakable. Her strength was failing and her body had become fragile in ways that humour and resolve could no longer conceal. The decline was no longer incremental; it was clearly accelerating.

And still, life insisted on proceeding.

Both my children were home with me, and it was my daughter's sixth birthday, so I decided to host a party for her. I don't know why; perhaps I was clinging to normalcy or perhaps I just needed *something* to continue as planned.

uMa insisted on attending the party, but the day became an exercise in vigilance for all of us. She could no longer manage much without assistance. Walking short distances was effortful, keeping food down was uncertain, and even breathing had become laboured. Every activity of daily living was difficult. She was vomiting and weak, so we spent most of the party arranging medical attention, monitoring symptoms, adjusting medication, and negotiating safety moment by moment.

By this point, the support structure around uMa had become fragile. My grandmother, who had lived with her, now required full-time care herself and was in the process of being moved to an old age home. Aunt Mfusi, uMa's closest friend, had stepped in where she could, as had domestic help when it was available, but there was no one there consistently, full time, every day. I could not move to her, so I needed to find a way for uMa to go home with me.

That week, she was admitted to hospital again. This time, the conversation changed.

"I will get her stable enough for you to fly," her doctor told me. "When you arrive, take her straight to hospital on the other side."

It was not certainty, and it was conditional, but it was permission.

Before we left for the airport, uMa asked for a moment alone with her own mother. She walked slowly into Gogo's bedroom and closed the door behind her. The rest of us waited quietly in the house. uMa and Gogo's relationship had always been complicated; loving in its own way, but also marked by years of tension and unspoken history.

They were in there for some time, and when the door finally opened, uMa stepped out quietly. The house had gone still. She did not say anything, but her eyes were filled with tears. We understood, without needing to ask, that something important had passed between them.

What followed was an extraordinary collaboration. uMa's treating team in KwaZulu-Natal coordinated with a group of doctors in Cape Town – clinicians who had never met her, who knew her only through reports and phone calls, but who were still willing to take on the risk. There was professional trust, and a shared commitment to continuity of care.

Against the odds, a plan formed.

uMa and I flew together. My siblings and other family stood at the airport watching us leave. Sis' Gugu held herself steady in the way caregivers often do when exhaustion and love sit side by side. Noma stood nearby, quiet and watchful. They waved as we moved through the departure gates.

None of us knew it then, but it would be the last time my sisters saw uMa walking and talking. They would speak to her by phone in the weeks that followed, but they would not see her in person again until the final days, by which time she could no longer respond. Mpe, who came to stay and help with her care, would have more time with her, but that afternoon none of us understood what we were witnessing

One phase was ending, but for uMa and me, something else was beginning.

For the first time in months, I did not have to worry from a distance. I did not have to imagine her dying alone, undiscovered for days. She was with me, contained, held within a system that could respond.

This was not a rescue, and it was not a perfect solution, but it was proximity, and that mattered enormously.

From that moment on, my and Ma's healing journey, such as it could be, truly began.

Reflection: Then and Now

I thought caregiving required physical presence, but this period taught me that coordination, advocacy, and vigilance are equally important forms of care, even if some don't see them.

Distance had magnified every fear, and while proximity did not remove the reality of what was happening, it changed the way we carried it.

Clinical Insight: Invisible Caregiving Labour

Administrative caregiving – like making calls, getting reports and coordinating various aspects – is cognitively taxing and rarely recognised. Caregivers often manage complex logistical systems while simultaneously navigating emotional strain. This invisible labour sometimes results in significant fatigue and contributes to caregiver burnout, even when the work is not visibly physical.

Recognising this form of caregiving is an essential part of supporting those who carry it.

Caregiver Takeaway

If your administrative caregiving feels invisible, take heart: it is no less real. Coordination, advocacy, and decision making are all forms of care. Bear in mind that exhaustion does not require witnesses to be valid.

6

From July 2015 – Held

When we arrived in Cape Town, we went straight to the hospital. Then we began again. New doctors. New rooms. New waiting areas that did not yet carry memory. We arrived carrying thick paper files, months of illness compressed into paper and ink, evidence of decisions that had been made elsewhere.

One oncologist stands out in my memory. He was older, measured. He read through uMa's file carefully before looking up at us.

"There isn't much more we can do," he said gently. "Our focus now is comfort."

There was no urgency in his voice. No attempt to soften the truth by obscuring it. He did not speak over uMa or around her, he spoke to us clearly and respectfully, without diminishing the moment. Something settled in that room.

Despite his pronouncement, we still consulted a nephrologist and additional clinicians, because some part of me still needed to test the edges of possibility. Hope had not disappeared; it had simply changed shape. And through it all, the doctors remained consistent: honest, present, and kind. They did not withdraw because cure was no longer an option; care continued.

At work, I was being held in a different way. My employer did not demand explanations, and my colleagues did not scrutinise my hours or question my absences. There were no subtle reminders about productivity or performance. There was trust – quiet, professional, and deeply humane. No one asked me to perform resilience, they just allowed me to work as I could, when I could. That, too, was care.

Among my inner circle was someone I had known long before this season. I had met Mam' Duduzile Mashalaba years earlier, in 2008, when we started work on the same day. I was newly qualified, just out of community service and still learning how to carry responsibility. She was already in her mid- to late forties, entering a new chapter as a clinical psychologist after many years of working as a nurse. We came into that space from different directions, but over time, a quiet connection formed, and I came to know her as Mam' Mashalaba. By the time Ma became ill, our friendship was already well established. Something changed in the next season, though; not the relationship itself, but rather what it was asked to hold.

Mam' Mashalaba understood, in ways I did not have to explain, what I was navigating. Her own experiences with grief and palliative care gave her a language for things I could not yet name. During that time, she called me every day. Not occasionally. Not only when things escalated. Every day.

Sometimes she spoke with the clarity of a nurse, practical, grounded, and attentive to detail. She guided me through aspects of care that felt overwhelming when I was standing in them as a daughter. Other times, she did not guide at all, she just listened.

She allowed me to speak without needing to organise my thoughts, and without redirecting me toward solutions. In a season when I was expected to manage, understand, and remain composed, she created a space where I did not have to do any of that. I did not have to be a clinician when I spoke with her; I could just be a daughter.

Looking back, I recognise this as a particular kind of care – not formal or structured, but deeply sustaining. She did not try to fix what could not be fixed, she simply remained present. Her presence carried me in ways that enabled me to bear everything else I was holding.

At home, the household reorganised itself around Ma's illness. Mpe had already come down to live with us, and my other siblings also remained actively involved, checking in, coordinating, and sharing the responsibility even when they could not be physically present. Decisions were discussed. Emotional weight was distributed. The burden no longer belonged to one person alone.

Friends checked in, showing up even when they didn't know what to say. Those who couldn't come in person messaged or called, and these small gestures reminded me that I still existed beyond the crisis at hand. Their care did not intrude on our situation; it accompanied us so we felt less isolated.

My husband was not physically present, but he was unwavering in his support. From a distance, he offered what he could financially and emotionally through reassurance, patience and kindness. There were no conditions attached and no resentment. He understood that this season demanded more than could be evenly distributed.

By then, the house was full in a way it had never been before. First there were my children, still young, still needing routine. Next there was my mother, fragile but still there, resting in the next room while life continued around her. Then there was my brother, steady and present, and finally my helper who kept daily life running as smoothly as was possible.

Layered over it all was a network of people – siblings, friends, colleagues, clinicians – quietly absorbing what none of us could have carried alone. This, I would come to understand, was what good palliative care looked like: not heroic interventions or dramatic gestures, but honesty, shared responsibility, and care that extended beyond the patient to the people who loved her.

uMa was not abandoned by medicine, and I was not abandoned by my employer, my siblings, my friends, or my husband. In a season defined by loss, we were all being held. Collectively, consistently, and without spectacle.

Reflection: Then and Now

Only later did I recognise how rare this convergence was. Support often fractures under prolonged strain. In our case, it expanded, not because the situation was easier than any other, but because the people around us chose to respond with generosity rather than fear.

Clinical Insight: Networks of Care

Effective palliative care extends beyond clinical teams. Family, work colleagues, friends, and partners (distant or otherwise) all form an essential ecosystem that sustains the caregivers. When these systems are acknowledged and supported, caregivers are better able to remain present and regulated.

Caring for the carer is never a single intervention; it is a networked response.

Caregiver Takeaway

If support is offered, accept it. You are not meant to do this alone, and care is strongest when it is shared.

7

July–August 2015 – Sacred Conversations

Once life slowed down enough, the talking began. Not all at once, though, and not dramatically. Our conversations emerged in the quiet spaces like late afternoons, evenings that stretched longer than they used to, and nights interrupted by pain or breathlessness. When urgency receded, words found room to settle.

uMa spoke first about her childhood – where she grew up, and the places that shaped her before illness ever touched her life. She told me about being raised by her grandfather, the man who had steadied her earliest years. She spoke of him with fondness and pride, recalling what he did for a living, how he carried himself, and the sense of safety he provided. These stories arrived gently, as if she were returning parts of herself to the world.

Then she spoke about my father, about their marriage and its failure. She shared how it had wounded her, and the ways she knew she had failed too. There was no rewriting of history, no justification, just ownership.

She spoke about decisions she had made. Some she stood by, and others she regretted deeply. She apologised for choices she was not proud of, for past hurts and moments she wished she could undo.

There is something profoundly disarming about being apologised to by a dying parent. It rearranges power. It dissolves old narratives. It invites forgiveness not as obligation, but as grace.

We planned her funeral together. Matter-of-factly. Carefully. With laughter when the absurdity of it crept in. It was not morbid, it was practical. She wanted things done a certain way, and I listened, writing things down. In planning her goodbye, she was still parenting, still guiding.

And then, we lived.

We hired a wheelchair and went shopping. We went on coffee dates. We claimed ordinary pleasures with intention. When she could not sleep, I stayed up with her. When pain came, I bathed her and rubbed her body, learning the geography of her discomfort. I became her hands.

uMa played with my children when she had enough breath, singing softly or telling them small stories before exhaustion returned. Even in decline, she found ways to mother, and to leave memory rather than absence.

There were moments of joy that surprised me. Moments of humour. Moments when we were not patient and caregiver, but simply two women sharing space. Amid these conversations, she remained a mother to the end.

We spoke about my second sister, Khossy, her pending lobola negotiations, and the future she would step into after my mother's absence. Ma wanted things done properly. Respectfully. In keeping with who we were. She wrote her umembeso list in preparation for the event. Not hurriedly, not fearfully, but deliberately. Item by item, she prepared for a ritual she knew she would not witness; it was a way of placing herself into a future she would miss. Culture, in that moment, became continuity.

uMa also worried aloud about the children she would be leaving behind. She spoke about my youngest sister, Noma, who was still at university at the time, young and finding her way while managing her own health challenges, including a severe visual impairment. uMa feared Noma's vulnerability in a world that would expect independence too quickly. Noma, teasingly known as my firstborn, had always needed a particular kind of advocacy. uMa wondered who would advocate for Noma when she was no longer there to do so instinctively. I had fought Noma's battles for as long as I could remember, and uMa had watched me do it, and had done the same in her own way. Now she was wondering aloud what would happen when she was no longer there to be part of that. Who would see Noma the way we saw her? Who would step in without being asked?

She worried about Mpe – about his sense of purpose, his dignity, his path forward. She was not judgemental, merely concerned; the quiet concern of a parent who knows how easily confidence can erode when opportunity stalls.

These were not conversations steeped in panic, they were careful, measured, loving.

In speaking about her children, uMa was not seeking reassurance. She was naming what mattered, ensuring that each child was still held in mind, still accounted for, still anchored in the family narrative even as her body weakened. She was not clinging to life; she was arranging what would outlive her.

We also spoke about dying, not in abstraction or as a euphemism; we simply named its inevitability. We discussed what to expect, when to seek help, and what signs would mean the end was nearing. The doctors were honest, and we absorbed the information side by side.

Sometimes, she cried.

"I am scared of dying," she would say. I never knew what to say in return. There are no words that can dissolve that fear without dishonesty. I did not offer certainty I did not possess, and I did not redirect her grief. I just stayed.

uMa was not religious, but she carried a rosary anyway. She prayed quietly, just in case there was something waiting on the other side. She prayed not from conviction, but from humility, from the instinctive human hope that death might not be the end of consciousness, only its transformation.

We spoke about death daily.

Not in despair, not in avoidance, but with openness. In doing so, we stripped it of some of its terror. Acceptance did not arrive as peace; it arrived as honesty.

In those weeks, we did not conquer death and we did not make sense of it. What we did was make space for everything that still wanted to be said. We made space for love, regret, fear, laughter, forgiveness.

We were not brave. We were present.

Reflection: Then and Now

At the time, I often saw these conversations with uMa as a responsibility – more things to remember, more things to carry forward. I did not yet understand that conversations could heal without fixing anything. Bearing witness became our shared language of love.

Now, I understand these conversations as trust.

By speaking these worries aloud, uMa was entrusting me with her unfinished concerns – not as burdens, but as evidence of love that refused to end abruptly. She was handing over guardianship, passing the torch rather than dropping a weight. I received it as both the heaviness of responsibility, and the honour of being trusted with everything she could no longer oversee herself.

Clinical Insight: What the Dying Carry – Fears and Concerns at End of Life

Parents who are dying often carry deep concerns for the children they are leaving behind. This is not a sign of anxiety or unfinished emotional business, it is a natural expression of love extending itself beyond the limits of a lifetime. When the dying are given space to name these concerns aloud, it allows them to feel heard, and those left behind to feel entrusted rather than burdened.

While this account reflects a daughter caring for her mother, these conversations are not unique to that relationship. A partner facing death may worry about the one they are leaving to navigate life alone. A sibling may fear being forgotten. A parent losing a child may grieve the future they had imagined. Whatever the relationship, the dying often carry unspoken concerns about those they love and creating space for those concerns to be voiced is one of the most profound gifts a caregiver can offer.

An end-of-life review is a natural process that supports emotional integration. These conversations can reduce existential distress for both the patient and caregiver.

For caregivers, hearing these worries can feel heavy, but they also offer a roadmap for honouring legacy through action.

Caregiver Takeaway

If your loved one speaks about who they are worried about, listen closely. These are not expressions of fear alone; they are acts of care – love stretching itself beyond the limits of a single lifetime.

You do not need the right words. Presence is enough.

8

August–September 2015 – The Final Weeks

UMa's body began to let go in ways that could no longer be managed or negotiated.

Her breathing changed first, becoming irregular, shallow at times, then laboured. She could no longer feed herself. Eating became difficult, then almost impossible. I noticed the smell of her urine changed, becoming sharp and unmistakable. It was a sign the doctors had told me to watch for.

They had prepared me well. At first, it brought clarity knowing what to look for and what each change might mean, but there were moments when knowledge did not translate into certainty.

I remember speaking to a colleague during that time, trying to make sense of when to act, and when to take uMa back to hospital. Her condition had always been severe, so the line between "manageable" and "critical" felt blurred.

"How do I know when it's time?" I asked.

She answered simply: "Take her in when she is uncomfortable."

It was a small sentence, but it shifted everything. Until then, I had been thinking in terms of treatment – when intervention was needed, and when something could be fixed or stabilised. But there was no cure anymore.

uMa was not going to hospital to get better; she was going for comfort, the very definition of palliative care. That understanding changed how I responded. It gave me permission to stop searching for turning points that no longer existed, and to start responding to what she was feeling, not just what I was observing.

When uMa's pain increased, they offered morphine. At first, it brought hallucinations, moments of confusion and restlessness. But it also brought sleep; longer stretches of rest than she had known in weeks. Comfort began to take precedence over clarity, and I learned to accept that trade-off.

uMa worried a lot about suffocating. The fluid in her lung required regular drainage, and the sensation of breathlessness frightened her deeply. The doctors reassured us gently but firmly: it would not be her lungs that took her life.

"It will be her kidneys," they said. "She will sleep more and more. She will linger. And then one day, she will not wake up." There was no cruelty in their words, only honesty.

One day, I recognised the change immediately: the smell the doctor had told me to watch for, the discomfort, the shift I could not explain but could also not ignore. uMa was restless, uncomfortable, no longer settling despite medication. Her body had entered a different phase, one that no amount of vigilance could reverse.

I called her doctor. There was no urgency in his tone, only certainty. He told me to bring her in.

On the way to hospital, uMa cried. She knew she was not going to make it out again. And so did I.

When we arrived, the doctor examined uMa quietly, then looked at me meaningfully.

"Prepare the family," he said. "This is it. Whoever needs to say goodbye should come now."

She was admitted on a Monday.

I phoned my siblings and told them plainly what was happening. Some thought I was exaggerating. That is the cost of distance. When you do not witness the daily changes, the truth feels abrupt. Detail is lost. Urgency is questioned.

By the Thursday they'd all arrived.

With them was my mother's cousin and her closest friend, Aunt Mfusi. Aunt Mfusi had been a constant presence in all our lives, but especially during times that my siblings and I were not around. She and uMa had been friends since they were young, and she stepped in when my siblings and I could not, visiting, checking in, and often driving uMa to chemotherapy appointments. In many ways, she had carried parts of the caregiving that we could not always be physically present for.

Her presence at the end felt right.

By the time they arrived, uMa had already been sleeping for two days. I stayed with her continuously, day and night. There was no conversation left, only presence.

Silence became our shared language. Steady, uninterrupted, and enough.

She did not speak again.

I watched her breathing slow.

Lengthen.

Pause.

The room had grown quieter in the last few days. Time stretched differently there.

When my siblings gathered, we stood around her bed and prayed over her. We thanked her. We told her we loved her. We gave her permission to rest, though none of us was ready to live without her.

On Sunday, 6 September 2015, she did.

She rested.

In peace.

Reflection: Then and Now

I once thought the end would feel chaotic. Instead, it felt deliberate, marked by signs, preparation, and quiet witnessing. Death did not arrive as a thief; it came as a closing.

Being prepared did not lessen the pain, but it spared us confusion and allowed us to remain present rather than panicked.

Clinical Insight: Recognising the Actively Dying Phase

In the final weeks of life, physiological changes often signal systemic shutdown: reduced appetite, altered breathing, renal failure, and prolonged sleep. Clear communication from clinicians empowers caregivers to respond with calm, dignity, and presence.

Preparing families for what to expect is not pessimism. It's compassion.

Caregiver Takeaway

If you are told that the end is near, trust the preparation you've been given. You do not need to fill the silence. Sitting with someone as they die is not passive, it is an act of profound care.

9

After

UMa was our only parent.

Our only constant.

Our only safety net.

We did not have a wide extended family to absorb the loss. There was no surplus of elders to step in, and no layered hierarchy of support to catch us when she fell away. When she died, what remained was us: siblings holding one another with uneven strength, learning in real time what it meant to live without the person who had anchored everything.

We tried to hold on to that.

Some days we did better than others.

After her death, we transported her body back to her home in Umzinto so that those who had loved her – family, friends, colleagues, neighbours – could say goodbye. She had been well known in her community, respected for her warmth and presence.

The turnout was large. Stories flowed easily, and laughter sat beside grief, as it often does when someone has lived fully. It was comforting to see how many lives she had touched, but it was also disorienting. When the rituals ended, the visitors left, and the noise softened, the reality returned unchanged: love from a community does not replace the loss of a mother.

It honours it, but it does not fill the space she occupied.

Our family home, uMa's home, became something else after that – an empty shell. It was difficult to visit, heavy with memory. Rooms still held her presence in ways that felt both tender and unbearable. There are houses you grieve not because they are empty, but because they remember too much. Ours became one of those.

We learned that grief does not move forward in a straight line.

It circles.

It revisits.

It resurfaces without warning.

There was no moment that we "got over" losing uMa, only moments when we learned how to carry the loss differently.

And still, here we are. Living, not because we are strong in the ways people like to celebrate, but because life insists on continuing even when it feels unjust.

We show up for one another imperfectly. We falter. We disagree – about opinions, about choices, about the small and large things that siblings have always disagreed about. And we repair our relationships again because the alternative is losing what little remains. We hold on to the small thread of family that remains because it is all we have – and because it matters.

uMa did not leave us prepared for her absence, no parent ever can, but she left us something else: honesty, love spoken aloud, forgiveness given and received, and the memory of being deeply seen in her final months.

That has not made life easier, but it has made it truer. Palliative care did not save uMa's life, but it gave us time, it gave us truth, and it gave us dignity. And in the end, that was enough.

This book does not close with peace.

It closes with presence.

With siblings still trying.

With a house that it hurts to enter.

With a life that continues carrying love forward, even when the source of that love is gone.

This is not an ending; it is what comes after love has nowhere left to go.

Reflection: Then and Now

I once believed grief would move forward. Instead, I discovered it circles – and teaches.

Clinical Insight: Grief After Caregiving

Caregiver grief is layered. It includes not only the loss of the person, but also the loss of role, structure, and identity.

After prolonged caregiving, individuals may experience a collapse of purpose alongside grief. This is not pathological; it is a natural response to the sudden absence of sustained responsibility and emotional attachment.

Grief after caregiving is often misunderstood and may be prolonged.

Supporting the caregiver during this phase is as important as supporting them during the active caregiving phase.

Caregiver Takeaway

If you are still grieving, you are not stuck, you are remembering.

AUTHOR'S NOTE

FOR CAREGIVERS

If you have found yourself in these pages, it is likely because you are caring for someone you love, or you are still carrying the weight of having done so.

Caregiving will ask more of you than you expect. It will blur roles, exhaust your reserves, and expose parts of yourself you did not know existed. You may feel strong one moment and undone the next. Both are true. Neither disqualifies you from being a good caregiver.

You do not need to say everything perfectly.

You do not need to be brave all the time.

You do not need to carry this alone.

If there is one thing I learned, it is this: presence matters more than certainty. Sitting with discomfort, staying when there are no solutions, and allowing yourself to be seen, these are acts of care, even when they feel inadequate.

When it ends, the world will not pause to acknowledge what you have lost. But you will know. Your body will know. Give yourself time to grieve not only the person you loved, but also the version of yourself that existed before this journey began.

If you are still in the middle of it: you are not failing.

If you are in the aftermath: you are not broken.

Whatever you may feel, you are responding normally to an extraordinary demand.

CLINICAL EPILOGUE

FOR HEALTHCARE PROFESSIONALS

Palliative care is not the absence of treatment, it is the presence of care.

Throughout this journey, what sustained my family was not intervention alone, but also communication – honest, compassionate, and consistent. We were blessed with clinicians who spoke clearly without removing hope, professionals who acknowledged the caregiver as part of the unit of care, and teams who prepared us for what was coming rather than shielding us from reality.

I cannot overstate what a difference this made.

When families are prepared, they panic less.

When caregivers are supported, they endure more safely.

When truth is delivered with kindness, trust is preserved.

Caregivers are often the unseen workforce of palliative care. They manage symptoms, coordinate services, absorb emotional distress, and make ethically complex decisions, often while holding jobs, families, and their own grief. Asking "How are you coping?" is not a courtesy, it is a clinical intervention.

Equally important is recognising moral distress in caregivers – the quiet suffering that arises when they know what is needed but are constrained by systems, timing, or circumstance. Naming this experience matters because it validates what cannot be fixed.

As healthcare professionals, our role does not end when curative options are exhausted. In many ways, that's when our role becomes more important. How we speak, how we prepare families, and how we hold uncertainty will shape how this story is remembered long after death.

Palliative care does not change outcomes, it changes experiences.

And that difference lasts a lifetime.

ACKNOWLEDGMENTS

This book was written in the quiet aftermath of profound loss and overwhelming care. It exists because many people held my family together when we could no longer hold ourselves.

I sincerely thank the doctors, nurses, and allied health professionals who practised palliative care with honesty, skill, and humanity, and who prepared us for what was coming rather than shielding us from it. Your words mattered more than you may ever know.

To my former colleagues and former employer, thank you for recognising that caregiving is real work, and for responding with trust rather than scrutiny. Your flexibility allowed me to remain both a professional and a daughter.

To my siblings, who shared the weight of loving and losing our only parent, thank you for standing with me, imperfectly and faithfully, when there was no one else to lean on.

To my brother, who moved into a house already heavy with grief and helped make it liveable again, your presence mattered.

To my friends, who checked in without demanding explanations, your quiet constancy carried me through more than you know.

To my husband, who held us from afar with patience, generosity, and unwavering support, thank you for understanding that love sometimes looks like absence without abandonment.

And finally, to my children, you lived alongside illness and loss with a grace that humbled me. You reminded me daily that life continues even in the shadow of goodbye.

ABOUT THE AUTHOR

Anothile Dolo is an occupational therapist based in South Africa, with professional experience spanning clinical practice, insurance disability claims assessments, medico-legal evaluations, and functional capacity evaluations. Her work has involved assessing patients' functional capacity and ability that leads to real life decisions that affect individuals, families, and systems of care.

Anothile has worked in public health, private practice, and insurance environments, including senior roles within disability claims management and medico-legal reporting. Her professional background has required her to navigate difficult ethical decisions and to sit with uncertainty while never losing sight of the long-term impact illness has on the people behind the files.

This book was written from her dual perspective as a clinician and as a daughter who cared for her terminally ill mother. While grounded in professional experience, *Caring for the Carer* is not a clinical text. It is a personal account of caregiving, loss, and palliative care as lived from the inside, informed by practice, but shaped by love.

Anothile lives in South Africa with her family.

www.ingramcontent.com/pod-product-compliance
Lightning Source LLC
LaVergne TN
LVHW100733061126
851857LV00011B/521
* 9 7 8 0 9 0 3 7 3 3 8 1 6 *